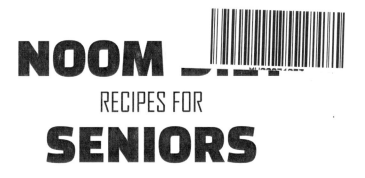

NOOM DIET
RECIPES FOR
SENIORS

A Delicious and Nutritious Diet Recipes for Seniors
to Boost Energy, Vitality and Long-Term Weight
Loss and Healthy Aging

MURPHY LAWSON

TABLE OF CONTENT

INTRODUCTION...9

UNDERSTANDING THE NOOM DIET PLAN............................11

What exactly is the Noom Diet Plan?.................................11

How does it Work? 12

- Green Foods:...13
- Yellow Foods: 13
- Red Foods:..13

The benefits of the Noom Diet Plan for seniors 14

Tailored to Seniors' Nutritional Needs: 14

Encourages Good Routines: 15

Flexible and Customizable: 15

Whole, Nutrient-Dense Foods:...15

Provided Coaching and Support: 16

THE NOOM DIET FOOD CATEGORIES...................................17

Understanding the colour-coded food categories 17

1.   Green Foods: 17

2.   Yellow Foods: 18

3.   Red Foods: 18

How to incorporate each food category into your diet.....19

Green Foods:..19

Yellow Foods:...19

Red Foods:...20

Tips for planning meals using the Noom food categories..21

Start with green foods: 21

Add yellow foods in moderation:............................. 21

Limit red foods:... 22

Plan your meals:... 22

Experiment with new recipes:.............................. 23

NOOM DIET RECIPES FOR SENIORS **24**

Breakfast Recipes... **24**

Veggie Omelette 24

Greek Yogurt Parfait... 25

Avocado Toast 26

Apple Cinnamon Oatmeal 27

Quinoa and Egg Breakfast Bowl 28

Peanut Butter Banana Smoothie.......................... 29

Spinach and Mushroom Frittata.......................... 30

Greek Yogurt Parfait... 33

Veggie and Cheese Frittata................................ 34

Chia Seed Pudding 35

Lunch Recipes **37**

Grilled Chicken Salad with Citrus Dressing 37

Lentil and Vegetable Soup................................. 39

Grilled Vegetable Wrap..................................... 40

Tuna Salad Lettuce Wraps................................. 41

Quinoa and Vegetable Stir Fry 43

Roasted Vegetable and Hummus Wrap 44

Chicken and Black Bean Salad 45

Lentil and Sweet Potato Salad 47

Greek Chicken Pita Pocket 48

Dinner Recipes **51**

Grilled Salmon with Asparagus and Brown Rice............. 51

Quinoa and Black Bean Stuffed Bell Peppers 52

Chickpea and Vegetable Stir-Fry 54

Grilled Salmon with Roasted Vegetables 56

Vegetarian Quinoa and Black Bean Chili 57

Baked Chicken Thighs with Sweet Potatoes and Brussels
Sprouts 59

Lemon Garlic Shrimp with Broccoli and Quinoa 60

Turkey and Vegetable Skillet 61

Baked Salmon with Asparagus and Quinoa 63

Snack Recipes **65**

Roasted Edamame: 65

Greek Yogurt and Berry Parfait: 66

Baked Zucchini Chips: 66

Apple Slices with Almond Butter: 68

Carrots and Hummus: 68

Cottage Cheese and Berries 69

Baked Apple Chips 70

Greek Yogurt and Granola 71

Apple Cinnamon Yogurt Parfait 71

Roasted Chickpeas 72

Dessert Recipes **74**

Banana Oatmeal Cookies 74

Berry and Yogurt Parfait 75

Baked Apples with Cinnamon and Almonds 76

Berry and Yogurt Parfait 77

Baked Apples with Cinnamon and Walnuts 78

Chocolate Banana Smoothie 79

Vanilla Chia Pudding 80

Peanut Butter Banana Bites 81

Baked Apple Slices 81

Chocolate Chia Pudding 83

MEAL PLANNING FOR THE NOOM DIET **84**

How to Plan Your Weekly Meals **84**

1.   Take stock of your Pantry and Refrigerator: 84

2.   Plan your Meals for the Week: 84

3.   Create a Grocery List: 85

4.   Shop for Groceries: 85

5.   Prepare your Ingredients: 85

Sample meal plans for seniors on the Noom Diet **86**

Week 1: 86

Week 2: 89

Week 3: 92

Week 4: 95

Tips for Grocery Shopping and Meal Prep **98**

Make a Grocery List: 98

Shop the Perimeter: 98

Buy in bulk: 99

Prep in Advance: 99

Use meal Prep Containers: 99

Don't be afraid to freeze: 99

Stay organized: 100

NOOM DIET SUCCESS TIPS FOR SENIORS **101**

Staying motivated on the Noom Diet **101**

Set achievable goals: 101

Find a support system: 101

Celebrate successes: 102

Keep it interesting: 102

Track progress: 102

Overcoming common challenges and obstacles 102

1.   Lack of motivation: 103

2.   Cravings: 103

3.   Eating out: 103

4.   Social pressure: 104

5.   Plateaus: 104

Lifestyle changes to support your weight loss goals 104

Regular Exercise: 105

Adequate sleep: 105

Stress management: 105

Mindful eating: 106

Hydration: 106

Conclusion 107

Appendix: Noom Diet Food List 108

Green Foods: 108

Yellow Foods: 108

Red Foods: 109

Glossary 110

Noom Coach: 110

Calorie Density: 110

Green Foods: 110

Yellow Foods: 110

Red Foods: 111

Portion Control: 111

Mindful Eating: 111

Meal Planning: 111

Meal Prep: 111

Plate Method: 112

INTRODUCTION

I want to start by saying thank you for choosing this book. I hope you found it insightful and helpful.

Our dietary demands alter as we age, making it more difficult to maintain a healthy weight and general health. That's where the Noom Diet comes in, providing elders with a flexible, long-term strategy to weight loss and improved health.

The Noom Diet plan, created by a group of behavioural psychologists, nutritionists, and personal trainers, emphasizes whole, nutrient-dense meals and encourages seniors to adopt lifestyle adjustments that support their weight reduction objectives. Seniors may make informed meal choices and remain on track with their weight reduction quest by utilizing a colour-coded system to categorize foods based on their calorie density and nutritional value.

Nutritionist Murphy Lawson presents a complete reference to the Noom Diet plan, designed exclusively for elders, in this Noom Diet Recipes for Seniors book. Murphy offers her knowledge and experience, providing ideas for meal planning, grocery shopping, and making healthy choices, as well as tasty, easy-to-prepare meals tailored to seniors' nutritional needs.

Whether you want to reduce weight, enhance your health, or simply eat healthier, the Noom Diet Recipes for Seniors book is a great place to start. This book will help you reach your health goals and feel your best by combining a flexible and sustainable approach to weight loss with professional assistance and delicious recipes. So, why delay? Begin your road to a healthier, happier self today by purchasing Noom Diet Recipes for Seniors.

CHAPTER ONE

UNDERSTANDING THE NOOM DIET PLAN

What exactly is the Noom Diet Plan?

The Noom diet plan is a versatile, long-term weight-loss strategy that promotes whole, nutrient-dense meals and supports lifestyle adjustments that are increasingly aware of the benefits of health goals. The approach employs a colour-coded system to categorize foods based on their calorie density and nutritional content, to assist consumers in making educated eating choices.

The Noom diet plan is tailored to each individual's preferences, with an emphasis on developing good habits and making long-term adjustments to assist weight reduction and general health. The plan includes a range of foods, such as fruits and vegetables, lean meats, and whole grains, and encourages people to make gradual, lasting adjustments to their eating habits rather than rigorous, unsustainable diets.

In addition to dietary categories, the Noom diet plan incorporates coaching and support via the Noom app, which gives individualized feedback, daily challenges, and educational tools to assist users in meeting their weight reduction objectives.

Ultimately, the Noom diet plan is intended to be a flexible and long-term strategy to weight loss and improved health, focusing on healthy behaviours and lifestyle adjustments rather than quick cures.

How does it Work?

The Noom diet plan employs a colour-coded system to classify foods depending on their calorie density and nutritional content. The objective is to assist individuals in making educated food choices and to generate long-term improvements in their eating patterns.

The following are the colour-coded food categories utilized in the Noom diet plan:

- **Green Foods:** Green vegetables are nutrient-dense, low-calorie foods that should comprise the majority of your diet. Fruits, vegetables, whole grains, and lean meats are among the examples.

- **Yellow Foods:** Provide moderate calories and should be taken in moderation. Lean meats, dairy, and some grains are examples.

- **Red Foods:** These are heavy in calories and poor in nutrients, and should be taken in moderation. Processed meals, sweets, and fatty meats are all examples.

Those on the Noom diet plan may build a healthy and long-lasting approach to weight loss and greater health by focusing on green foods and including yellow and red foods in moderation. Furthermore, the Noom app offers individualized coaching and support, such as daily challenges, progress monitoring, and educational materials, to assist users in staying on track with their objectives and making long-term lifestyle changes.

The Noom diet plan also emphasizes the significance of making progressive, long-term adjustments to one's eating habits and lifestyle, rather than rigorous, short-term diets. Individuals can build long-term habits that support their weight reduction and general health objectives by making incremental, attainable adjustments over time.

The benefits of the Noom Diet Plan for seniors
For seniors wishing to enhance their health and lose weight, the Noom diet plan has various advantages. Following are some of the main advantages:

Tailored to Seniors' Nutritional Needs: The Noom diet plan is particularly developed to fulfil the nutritional demands of elders, who may have more varied dietary needs than younger ones. The plan emphasizes full, nutrient-dense meals that supply seniors with the vitamins, minerals, and other nutrients they require to be healthy.

Encourages Good Routines: The Noom diet plan focuses on building long-term lifestyle changes that assist weight loss and improved health. The initiative encourages seniors to build healthy behaviours including meal planning, grocery shopping, and making educated food choices.

Flexible and Customizable: The Noom diet plan is meant to be adaptable and changeable to accommodate the demands of each individual. Rather than adhering to stringent and unsustainable diets, seniors can pick from a range of healthful foods and make modest, lasting modifications to their eating patterns.

Whole, Nutrient-Dense Foods: The Noom diet plan prioritizes entire, nutrient-dense foods including fruits, vegetables, lean meats, and whole grains. These meals supply seniors with the vitamins, minerals, and other nutrients they require to be healthy.

Provided Coaching and Support: Through the Noom app, which includes daily challenges, progress monitoring, and educational materials for elders. This assistance can help seniors keep on track with their weight reduction and general health objectives, as well as achieve long-term lifestyle adjustments.

Generally, the Noom diet plan has many advantages for seniors who want to enhance their health and reduce weight. Seniors may achieve lasting lifestyle changes that promote long-term health and wellness by prioritizing good behaviours, whole, nutrient-dense meals, and individualized coaching and support.

CHAPTER TWO

THE NOOM DIET FOOD CATEGORIES

Understanding the colour-coded food categories

The Noom diet plan uses a colour-coded system to categorize foods based on their calorie density and nutritional value. The goal of this system is to help individuals make informed choices about what they eat and to create sustainable changes to their eating habits over time.

Here are the colour-coded food categories used in the Noom diet plan:

1. **Green Foods:** These are nutrient-dense, low-calorie foods that should make up the bulk of your diet. Examples include fruits, vegetables, whole grains, and lean proteins. These foods are high in fibre and other important nutrients, and they can help you feel full and satisfied without consuming too many calories.

2. **Yellow Foods:** These are moderate-calorie foods that should be consumed in moderation. Examples include lean meats, dairy, and some grains. While these foods are higher in calories than green foods, they still provide important nutrients and can be part of a healthy diet in moderation.

3. **Red Foods:** These are high-calorie, low-nutrient foods that should be consumed in limited quantities. Examples include processed foods, sweets, and fatty meats. While these foods can be enjoyed occasionally, they should not make up a large part of your diet. Consuming too many red foods can lead to weight gain and other health problems.

By focusing on green foods and incorporating yellow and red foods in moderation, individuals on the Noom diet plan can create a balanced and sustainable approach to weight loss and better health. The goal is to make healthy choices most of the time, while still allowing for flexibility and enjoyment in your eating habits.

How to incorporate each food category into your diet

Incorporating each food category into your diet on the Noom diet plan is easy with the colour-coded system. Here are some tips for incorporating each food category into your diet:

Green Foods: Aim to make green foods the bulk of your diet. Choose a variety of fruits, vegetables, whole grains, and lean proteins to ensure that you're getting a wide range of important nutrients. Make sure to include at least one serving of green foods with every meal and snack.

Yellow Foods: Incorporate yellow foods in moderation. Choose lean meats, dairy, and grains that provide important nutrients without adding too many calories to your diet. Aim to include a serving or two of yellow foods each day.

Red Foods: Limit your consumption of red foods. Choose to enjoy these foods occasionally and in small quantities. Be mindful of portion sizes and try to choose healthier alternatives whenever possible.

Here are some specific examples of how to incorporate each food category into your diet:

Green foods: Add a handful of spinach or kale to your morning smoothie, enjoy a side salad with your lunch, and roast a variety of vegetables to serve with dinner.

Yellow foods: Choose lean proteins such as grilled chicken or fish for your main dish, add a serving of whole-grain pasta to your dinner, and enjoy a serving of Greek yoghurt with fresh berries as a snack.

Red foods: Indulge in a small serving of dark chocolate or a scoop of ice cream for dessert, enjoy a few chips with guacamole as a snack, and choose a small serving of fries as a side dish when eating out.

By incorporating a variety of foods from each colour category into your diet, you can create a balanced and sustainable approach to eating on the Noom diet plan.

Tips for planning meals using the Noom food categories

Planning meals using the Noom food categories can be a helpful way to ensure that you're getting a balanced and nutritious diet while following the Noom diet plan. Here are some tips for planning meals using the colour-coded food categories:

Start with green foods: Aim to make green foods the foundation of your meal. Start by choosing a variety of fruits and vegetables that you enjoy and build your meal around them. For example, you might create a big salad with lots of colourful vegetables and top it with a lean protein like grilled chicken or tofu.

Add yellow foods in moderation: Once you have your base of green foods, you can add some yellow foods in moderation. Choose lean proteins like fish or turkey breast, whole grains like brown rice or quinoa, and low-fat dairy products like Greek yoghurt or skim milk. Aim to include a serving or two of yellow foods with each meal.

Limit red foods: While it's okay to enjoy red foods occasionally, it's important to keep them in moderation. Limit your intake of high-calorie, low-nutrient foods like processed snacks, sugary drinks, and fatty meats. When you do indulge in red foods, try to choose healthier options like dark chocolate or baked sweet potato fries.

Plan your meals: To make meal planning easier, try planning your meals. This will help you ensure that you're getting a balanced diet and can make it easier to stick to your goals. Try using a meal planning app or creating a weekly menu to help you stay on track.

Experiment with new recipes: To keep things interesting, try experimenting with new recipes that incorporate a variety of green, yellow, and red foods. Look for healthy recipes that include lots of colourful vegetables, lean proteins, and whole grains. This can help you stay motivated and excited about your meals.

By following these tips and incorporating a variety of foods from each colour category into your meals, you can create a healthy and balanced diet that supports your weight loss and overall health goals on the Noom diet plan.

CHAPTER THREE

NOOM DIET RECIPES FOR SENIORS

Breakfast Recipes

Here are some healthy breakfast recipes that incorporate the Noom diet principles for seniors:

Veggie Omelette

Ingredients:

2 large eggs

1/2 cup chopped veggies (such as bell peppers, onions, mushrooms, and spinach)

1/4 cup shredded low-fat cheese

Salt and pepper to taste

1 teaspoon olive oil

Instructions:

In a small bowl, whisk together the eggs with salt and pepper.

Heat olive oil in a nonstick skillet over medium heat.

Add the chopped veggies and sauté until tender.

Pour the egg mixture into the skillet and let it cook until it begins to set.

Sprinkle the shredded cheese over half of the omelette.

Use a spatula to fold the omelette in half and let it cook for another minute or until the cheese is melted.

Serve hot with a side of fruit.

Nutritional Information (per serving):

Calories: 276

Protein: 22g

Fat: 19g

Carbs: 5g

Fibre: 1g

Greek Yogurt Parfait

Ingredients:

1 cup plain Greek yoghurt

1/2 cup mixed berries (such as strawberries, blueberries, and raspberries)

1/4 cup low-fat granola

1 tablespoon honey

Instructions:

In a bowl, mix the Greek yoghurt and honey until well combined.

Layer the yoghurt mixture, mixed berries, and granola in a glass or jar.

Repeat the layers until all ingredients are used up.

Serve immediately.

Nutritional Information (per serving):

Calories: 288

Protein: 20g

Fat: 5g

Carbs: 43g

Fibre: 6g

Avocado Toast

Ingredients:

1 slice of whole-grain bread

1/2 ripe avocado, mashed

1 small tomato, sliced

Salt and pepper to taste

1 teaspoon olive oil

Instructions:

Toast the bread until crispy.

Spread the mashed avocado on top of the toast.

Arrange the sliced tomato on top of the avocado.

Drizzle with olive oil and sprinkle with salt and pepper. Serve immediately.

Nutritional Information (per serving):

Calories: 215

Protein: 5g

Fat: 15g

Carbs: 18g

Fibre: 7g

Apple Cinnamon Oatmeal

Ingredients:

1/2 cup old-fashioned oats

1 cup unsweetened almond milk

1 small apple, chopped

1/4 teaspoon ground cinnamon

1 tablespoon chopped walnuts

1 teaspoon honey (optional)

Instructions:

In a small saucepan, bring the almond milk to a boil.

Add the oats and chopped apple to the saucepan.

Reduce the heat and let the oats cook for 5-7 minutes, stirring occasionally.

Remove from heat and stir in the cinnamon.

Top with chopped walnuts and a drizzle of honey, if desired.

Serve hot.

Nutritional Information (per serving):

Calories: 300

Protein: 9g

Fat: 10g

Carbs: 45g

Fibre: 8g

Quinoa and Egg Breakfast Bowl

Ingredients:

1/2 cup cooked quinoa

1 large egg

1/4 cup chopped veggies (such as zucchini, bell peppers, and onions)

1 teaspoon olive oil

Salt and pepper to taste

1 tablespoon chopped fresh parsley

Instructions:

Heat olive oil in a nonstick skillet over medium heat.

Add the chopped veggies and sauté until tender.

Crack the egg into the skillet and let it cook until the whites are set and the yolk is still runny.

In a bowl, combine the cooked quinoa with the cooked veggies.

Top with the cooked egg.

Season with salt and pepper to taste.

Garnish with chopped fresh parsley.

Serve immediately.

Nutritional Information:

Calories: 330

Protein: 18g

Fat: 16g

Carbs: 29g

Fibre: 5g

Peanut Butter Banana Smoothie

Ingredients:

1 medium banana, frozen

1 tablespoon natural peanut butter

1/2 cup unsweetened almond milk

1/2 cup plain Greek yoghurt

1/2 teaspoon vanilla extract

1/4 teaspoon ground cinnamon

1 tablespoon chia seeds (optional)

Instructions:

Add the frozen banana, peanut butter, almond milk, Greek yoghurt, vanilla extract, and cinnamon to a blender.

Blend until smooth and creamy.

If desired, stir in the chia seeds.

Serve immediately.

Nutritional Information (per serving):

Calories: 305

Protein: 20g

Fat: 11g

Carbs: 36g

Fibre: 8g

Spinach and Mushroom Frittata

Ingredients:

4 large eggs

1/4 cup unsweetened almond milk

1/2 cup chopped spinach

1/2 cup sliced mushrooms

1/4 cup shredded low-fat cheese

Salt and pepper to taste

1 teaspoon olive oil

Instructions:

In a small bowl, whisk together the eggs with almond milk, salt, and pepper.

Heat olive oil in a nonstick skillet over medium heat.

Add the chopped spinach and sliced mushrooms to the skillet and sauté until tender.

Pour the egg mixture into the skillet and let it cook until it begins to set.

Sprinkle the shredded cheese over the top of the frittata.

Heat a non-stick pan over medium heat and add the egg mixture. Cook until the edges start to set, then use a spatula to gently lift and fold the edges towards the centre of the pan, allowing the uncooked eggs to flow underneath. Continue cooking until the eggs are set but still slightly moist on top.

Remove the pan from the heat and sprinkle the top with the chopped scallions and freshly ground black pepper. Use the spatula to fold the omelette in half and slide it onto a plate.

Serve hot with a side of whole grain toast and sliced avocado for a delicious and satisfying breakfast that is packed with protein, healthy fats, and fibre.

Nutrition Information per serving:

Calories: 280

Protein: 20g

Fat: 19g

Carbohydrates: 8g

Fibre: 2g

Sugar: 2g

Sodium: 465mg

Greek Yogurt Parfait

Ingredients:

1 cup plain Greek yoghurt

1/2 cup mixed berries (strawberries, blueberries, raspberries)

1/4 cup chopped nuts (almonds, walnuts, pecans)

1 tbsp honey

Instructions:

In a small bowl, mix the Greek yoghurt and honey.

In a separate bowl, mix the mixed berries.

In a serving glass, layer the Greek yoghurt mixture, mixed berries, and chopped nuts.

Repeat the layers until the glass is filled to the top.

Serve chilled.

Nutrition Information per serving:

Calories: 370

Protein: 20g

Fat: 23g

Carbohydrates: 25g

Fibre: 4g

Sugar: 19g

Sodium: 70mg

Veggie and Cheese Frittata

Ingredients:

4 large eggs

1/4 cup milk

1/4 cup chopped onions

1/4 cup chopped bell peppers

1/2 cup chopped spinach

1/4 cup shredded cheddar cheese

Salt and pepper to taste

1 tbsp olive oil

Instructions:

Preheat the oven to 375°F.

In a bowl, whisk together the eggs and milk. Add salt and pepper to taste.

In an oven-safe skillet, heat the olive oil over medium heat.

Add the onions and bell peppers and cook until soft.

Add the chopped spinach and cook until wilted.

Pour the egg mixture over the vegetables and sprinkle with shredded cheddar cheese.

Bake in the oven for 10-12 minutes or until the eggs are set.

Remove from the oven and let it cool for a few minutes.

Slice into wedges and serve hot.

Nutrition Information per serving:

Calories: 280

Protein: 17g

Fat: 20g

Carbohydrates: 5g

Fibre: 1g

Sugar: 2g

Sodium: 320mg

Chia Seed Pudding

Ingredients:

1/4 cup chia seeds

1 cup unsweetened almond milk

1/2 tsp vanilla extract

1 tbsp honey

1/4 cup mixed berries (strawberries, blueberries, raspberries)

Instructions:

In a jar, mix the chia seeds, almond milk, vanilla extract, and honey.

Cover the jar and refrigerate overnight or for at least 4 hours.

Before serving, give the chia seed pudding a good stir.

Top with mixed berries and serve chilled.

Nutrition Information per serving:

Calories: 230

Protein: 6g

Fat: 11g

Carbohydrates: 28g

Fibre: 12g

Sugar: 12g

Sodium: 110mg

These breakfast recipes are packed with nutrient-dense ingredients that provide sustained energy throughout the day, and they all fit within the Noom diet principles for seniors.

Lunch Recipes

Here is a delicious and healthy lunch recipe for seniors following the Noom diet:

Grilled Chicken Salad with Citrus Dressing

Ingredients:

2 cups mixed greens

1 grilled chicken breast, sliced

1/2 avocado, sliced

1/2 cup cherry tomatoes, halved

1/4 cup chopped red onion

1/4 cup crumbled feta cheese

1 tbsp chopped fresh parsley

Salt and pepper to taste

For the dressing:

2 tbsp freshly squeezed orange juice

2 tbsp freshly squeezed lemon juice

1 tbsp honey

1/4 cup olive oil

Salt and pepper to taste

Instructions:

In a large bowl, mix the mixed greens, grilled chicken breast, avocado, cherry tomatoes, and red onion.

In a small bowl, whisk together the orange juice, lemon juice, honey, olive oil, salt, and pepper to make the dressing.

Drizzle the dressing over the salad and toss to coat.

Top with crumbled feta cheese and chopped parsley.

Serve chilled.

Nutrition Information per serving:

Calories: 450

Protein: 25g

Fat: 34g

Carbohydrates: 16g

Fibre: 7g

Sugar: 8g

Sodium: 320mg

Lentil and Vegetable Soup

Ingredients:

1 cup brown lentils, rinsed and drained

1 onion, chopped

2 carrots, chopped

2 celery stalks, chopped

1 zucchini, chopped

3 cloves garlic, minced

6 cups vegetable broth

1 tsp dried oregano

1/2 tsp dried thyme

Salt and pepper to taste

Instructions:

In a large pot, sauté the onion, carrot, and celery until the onion is translucent.

Add the garlic, lentils, vegetable broth, oregano, thyme, salt, and pepper.

Bring to a boil and then reduce heat to a simmer. Cook for 20 minutes.

Add the chopped zucchini and cook for an additional 10-15 minutes, or until the lentils are tender.

Serve hot.

Nutrition Information per serving:

Calories: 240

Protein: 16g

Fat: 1g

Carbohydrates: 44g

Fibre: 16g

Sugar: 7g

Sodium: 890mg

Grilled Vegetable Wrap

Ingredients:

1 whole wheat wrap

1/2 cup mixed grilled vegetables (such as bell peppers, zucchini, and eggplant)

1/4 cup hummus

1/4 cup crumbled feta cheese

Salt and pepper to taste

Instructions:

Lay the whole wheat wrap flat and spread hummus over the centre.

Add the mixed grilled vegetables and crumbled feta cheese.

Sprinkle with salt and pepper to taste.

Roll the wrap tightly and slice it in half.

Serve at room temperature.

Nutrition Information per serving:

Calories: 310

Protein: 12g

Fat: 12g

Carbohydrates: 39g

Fibre: 7g

Sugar: 5g

Sodium: 720mg

Tuna Salad Lettuce Wraps

Ingredients:

1 can tuna, drained and flaked

1/4 cup chopped celery

1/4 cup chopped red onion

2 tbsp plain Greek yoghurt

1 tbsp Dijon mustard

Salt and pepper to taste

4 large lettuce leaves

Instructions:

In a medium bowl, mix the tuna, celery, red onion, Greek yoghurt, Dijon mustard, salt, and pepper.

Lay out the large lettuce leaves and spoon the tuna mixture into each one.

Roll the lettuce leaves around the tuna mixture to create a wrap.

Serve cold.

Nutrition Information per serving:

Calories: 140

Protein: 18g

Fat: 3g

Carbohydrates: 8g

Fibre: 2g

Sugar: 4g

Sodium: 450mg

Quinoa and Vegetable Stir Fry

Ingredients:

1 cup quinoa

2 cups water

1 tbsp olive oil

1 onion, chopped

2 garlic cloves, minced

1 red bell pepper, sliced

1 yellow bell pepper, sliced

2 cups broccoli florets

2 tbsp soy sauce

Salt and pepper to taste

Instructions:

Rinse quinoa thoroughly and cook according to package directions.

In a large pan, heat olive oil over medium-high heat.

Add onion and garlic and cook for 2-3 minutes.

Add bell peppers and broccoli and cook for another 5-7 minutes.

Add cooked quinoa to the pan and mix well.

Drizzle soy sauce over the mixture and season with salt and pepper.

Serve hot.

Nutrition Information per serving:

Calories: 300

Protein: 10g

Fat: 7g

Carbohydrates: 50g

Fibre: 8g

Sugar: 8g

Sodium: 650mg

Roasted Vegetable and Hummus Wrap

Ingredients:

1 whole wheat wrap

1/4 cup hummus

1/2 cup roasted vegetables (such as sweet potato, cauliflower, and Brussels sprouts)

1/4 cup crumbled feta cheese

Salt and pepper to taste

Instructions:

Lay the whole wheat wrap flat and spread hummus over the centre.

Add the roasted vegetables and crumbled feta cheese.

Sprinkle with salt and pepper to taste.

Roll the wrap tightly and slice it in half.

Serve at room temperature.

Nutrition Information per serving:

Calories: 320

Protein: 11g

Fat: 10g

Carbohydrates: 46g

Fibre: 9g

Sugar: 6g

Sodium: 610mg

Chicken and Black Bean Salad

Ingredients:

1 boneless, skinless chicken breast, cooked and shredded

1 can black beans, rinsed and drained

1/2 red onion, chopped

1/2 red bell pepper, chopped

1/2 cup cherry tomatoes, halved

1 avocado, diced

1 lime, juiced

1 tbsp olive oil

Salt and pepper to taste

Instructions:

In a large bowl, mix the shredded chicken, black beans, red onion, red bell pepper, cherry tomatoes, and avocado.

In a small bowl, whisk together the lime juice and olive oil.

Drizzle the dressing over the salad and season with salt and pepper.

Serve cold.

Nutrition Information per serving:

Calories: 420

Protein: 29g

Fat: 19g

Carbohydrates: 37g

Fibre: 14g

Sugar: 4g

Sodium: 420mg

Lentil and Sweet Potato Salad

Ingredients:

1 sweet potato, peeled and chopped

1 tbsp olive oil

Salt and pepper to taste

1 cup cooked lentils

1/4 cup chopped red onion

1/4 cup crumbled feta cheese

1/4 cup chopped fresh parsley

1 lemon, juiced

Instructions:

Preheat the oven to 400°F (200°C).

In a small bowl, whisk together olive oil, lemon juice, honey, and Dijon mustard. Drizzle the dressing over the salad and toss to combine.

Serve immediately or store in an airtight container in the refrigerator for up to 3 days.

Enjoy your delicious and nutritious lentil and sweet potato salad as a satisfying and filling lunch!

Nutrition information per serving:

Calories: 380

Protein: 14g

Fat: 12g

Carbohydrates: 59g

Fibre: 13g

Greek Chicken Pita Pocket

Ingredients:

4 whole wheat pita pockets

1 pound boneless, skinless chicken breast, sliced into thin strips

1 teaspoon dried oregano

1 teaspoon dried basil

1 teaspoon garlic powder

1/4 teaspoon salt

1/4 teaspoon black pepper

2 tablespoons olive oil

1/2 cup diced cucumber

1/2 cup diced tomato

1/4 cup crumbled feta cheese

1/4 cup plain Greek yoghurt

Juice of 1/2 lemon

Instructions:

In a small bowl, mix oregano, basil, garlic powder, salt, and black pepper.

Heat olive oil in a large skillet over medium heat. Add chicken and sprinkle with the spice mixture. Cook for 6-8 minutes, or until chicken is cooked through and no longer pink.

In a separate bowl, combine cucumber, tomato, feta cheese, Greek yoghurt, and lemon juice.

Warm the pita pockets in the microwave or oven for 10-15 seconds.

Stuff each pita pocket with the chicken and vegetable mixture.

Serve immediately or store in an airtight container in the refrigerator for up to 2 days.

Enjoy your tasty and protein-packed Greek chicken pita pockets for a healthy and satisfying lunch!

Nutrition information per serving:

Calories: 400

Protein: 35g

Fat: 13g

Carbohydrates: 38g

Fibre: 6g

Dinner Recipes

Here are some healthy and delicious Noom diet dinner recipes for seniors:

Grilled Salmon with Asparagus and Brown Rice

Ingredients:

4 (4-ounce) salmon fillets

1 pound asparagus, trimmed

1 tablespoon olive oil

Salt and black pepper to taste

2 cups cooked brown rice

Lemon wedges for serving

Instructions:

Preheat the grill to medium-high heat.

Brush salmon and asparagus with olive oil and season with salt and black pepper.

Place salmon and asparagus on the grill and cook for 4-5 minutes per side, or until salmon is cooked through and asparagus is tender.

Serve salmon and asparagus with brown rice and lemon wedges.

Enjoy your delicious and nutritious grilled salmon with asparagus and brown rice for a healthy and satisfying dinner!

Nutrition information per serving:

Calories: 400

Protein: 32g

Fat: 18g

Carbohydrates: 28g

Fibre: 5g

Quinoa and Black Bean Stuffed Bell Peppers

Ingredients:

4 large bell peppers, halved and seeded

1 cup cooked quinoa

1 can (15 ounces) of black beans, rinsed and drained

1/2 cup chopped onion

1/2 cup chopped tomato

1/4 cup chopped cilantro

1 tablespoon olive oil

1 teaspoon ground cumin

1/2 teaspoon chilli powder

1/4 teaspoon salt

1/4 teaspoon black pepper

Instructions:

Preheat oven to 375°F.

In a large bowl, mix cooked quinoa, black beans, onion, tomato, cilantro, olive oil, cumin, chilli powder, salt, and black pepper.

Place bell pepper halves in a baking dish and fill each half with the quinoa and black bean mixture.

Cover the dish with foil and bake for 30-35 minutes, or until bell peppers are tender.

Remove from the oven and let cool for a few minutes before serving.

Enjoy your flavorful and protein-packed quinoa and black bean-stuffed bell peppers for a satisfying and healthy dinner!

Nutrition information per serving (2 stuffed pepper halves):

Calories: 350

Protein: 16g

Fat: 6g

Carbohydrates: 64g

Fibre: 16g

Chickpea and Vegetable Stir-Fry

Ingredients:

1 can (15 ounces) chickpeas, rinsed and drained

2 cups mixed vegetables (such as bell pepper, zucchini, onion, and carrot), chopped

2 cloves garlic, minced

1 teaspoon grated ginger

1 tablespoon soy sauce

1 tablespoon honey

1 tablespoon cornstarch

1 tablespoon olive oil

Cooked brown rice for serving

Instructions:

In a small bowl, whisk together soy sauce, honey, and cornstarch.

Heat olive oil in a large skillet or wok over medium-high heat. Add garlic and ginger and stir-fry for 30 seconds.

Add mixed vegetables to the skillet and stir-fry for 3-4 minutes, or until vegetables are tender-crisp.

Add chickpeas and stir-fry for 1-2 minutes, or until chickpeas are heated through.

Pour the soy sauce mixture into the skillet and stir-fry for 1-2 minutes.

Nutrition Information:

Calories: 359

Fat: 9g

Carbohydrates: 55g

Fibre: 11g // Protein: 16g

This recipe is a great source of protein, fibre, and complex carbohydrates. Chickpeas provide a vegetarian source of protein, while vegetables provide a variety of nutrients and fibre. Brown rice provides complex carbohydrates for sustained energy. Overall, this is a healthy and satisfying meal that is perfect for the Noom diet plan.

Grilled Salmon with Roasted Vegetables
Ingredients:

4 salmon fillets

Salt and pepper

1 bunch of asparagus, trimmed

2 bell peppers, sliced

2 zucchini, sliced

2 cloves garlic, minced

1 tbsp olive oil

1 tsp dried basil

1 tsp dried oregano

Instructions:

Preheat the grill to medium-high heat.

Season salmon fillets with salt and pepper.

Grill salmon for 5-7 minutes per side, or until cooked through.

In a separate bowl, toss asparagus, bell peppers, zucchini, garlic, olive oil, basil, and oregano together.

Spread the vegetables on a baking sheet and roast at 400°F for 20-25 minutes, or until vegetables are tender and slightly charred.

Serve grilled salmon with roasted vegetables.

Nutritional Information:

Calories: 334

Fat: 16g

Carbohydrates: 14g

Fibre: 5g

Protein: 33g

This recipe is a great source of protein and healthy fats from the salmon, as well as fibre and nutrients from the roasted vegetables.

Vegetarian Quinoa and Black Bean Chili

Ingredients:

1 cup quinoa, cooked

1 onion, diced

2 cloves garlic, minced

1 red bell pepper, diced

1 green bell pepper, diced

2 cans black beans, drained and rinsed

1 can dice tomatoes

1 tbsp chilli powder

1 tsp ground cumin

Salt and pepper to taste

Fresh cilantro, chopped

Instructions:

In a large pot, sauté onions, garlic, and bell peppers until soft.

Add canned black beans, diced tomatoes, chilli powder, and cumin to the pot.

Add cooked quinoa to the pot and stir to combine.

Let the chilli simmer for 15-20 minutes, or until heated through.

Season with salt and pepper to taste.

Serve with fresh cilantro on top.

Nutritional Information:

Calories: 294

Fat: 2g

Carbohydrates: 55g

Fibre: 16g

Protein: 16g

This recipe is a great source of plant-based protein, fibre, and complex carbohydrates, making it a filling and nutritious option for dinner.

Baked Chicken Thighs with Sweet Potatoes and Brussels Sprouts

Ingredients:

4 chicken thighs

Salt and pepper

2 sweet potatoes, peeled and cubed

1 lb Brussels sprouts, trimmed and halved

2 tbsp olive oil

1 tbsp honey

1 tbsp Dijon mustard

1 tsp dried thyme

Instructions:

Preheat oven to 425°F.

Season chicken thighs with salt and pepper.

Toss sweet potatoes and Brussels sprouts with olive oil, salt, and pepper.

Arrange chicken and vegetables on a baking sheet.

In a small bowl, whisk together honey, Dijon mustard, and dried thyme.

Brush the honey mustard mixture over the chicken.

Bake for 30-35 minutes, or until chicken is cooked through and vegetables are tender.

Nutritional Information:

Calories: 346

Fat: 17g

Carbohydrates: 25g

Fibre: 6g

Protein: 27

Lemon Garlic Shrimp with Broccoli and Quinoa

Ingredients:

1 lb. large shrimp, peeled and deveined

1 head broccoli, cut into florets

1 cup cooked quinoa

2 tbsp. olive oil

4 cloves garlic, minced

1 lemon, juiced and zested

Salt and pepper, to taste

Instructions:

Preheat the oven to 400°F.

In a large bowl, toss the shrimp, broccoli, olive oil, garlic, lemon zest, salt, and pepper together.

Spread the mixture on a baking sheet and roast for 12-15 minutes or until the shrimp is pink and cooked through.

Serve with cooked quinoa and a drizzle of lemon juice.

Nutritional Information:

Calories: 325

Protein: 32g

Fat: 12g

Carbohydrates: 24g

Fibre: 5g

Sugar: 3g

Sodium: 245mg

Turkey and Vegetable Skillet

Ingredients:

1 lb. ground turkey

1 red bell pepper, sliced

1 zucchini, sliced

1 yellow squash, sliced

1 onion, sliced

2 cloves garlic, minced

2 tbsp. olive oil

1 tsp. dried oregano

Salt and pepper, to taste

Instructions:

In a large skillet, heat the olive oil over medium-high heat.

Add the ground turkey and cook until browned and cooked through.

Add the bell pepper, zucchini, squash, onion, garlic, oregano, salt, and pepper to the skillet and cook until the vegetables are tender about 10 minutes.

Serve hot.

Nutritional Information:

Calories: 275

Protein: 29g

Fat: 13g

Carbohydrates: 10g

Fibre: 3g

Sugar: 5g

Sodium: 135mg

Baked Salmon with Asparagus and Quinoa

Ingredients:

4 salmon fillets

1 lb. asparagus, trimmed

1 cup cooked quinoa

2 tbsp. olive oil

2 cloves garlic, minced

1 lemon, sliced

Salt and pepper, to taste

Instructions:

Preheat the oven to 400°F.

In a large bowl, toss the asparagus, olive oil, garlic, salt, and pepper together.

Place the salmon fillets and asparagus on a baking sheet and top with lemon slices.

Bake for 12-15 minutes or until the salmon is cooked through.

Serve with cooked quinoa.

Nutritional Information:

Calories: 375

Protein: 37g

Fat: 17g

Carbohydrates: 19g

Fibre: 5g

Sugar: 2g

Sodium: 140mg

Snack Recipes

Here are Ten Noom diet snack recipes for seniors:

Roasted Edamame:

Ingredients:

1 cup of shelled edamame

1 tsp olive oil

Salt and pepper to taste

Instructions:

Preheat oven to 375°F (190°C).

Toss edamame with olive oil, salt, and pepper.

Spread the edamame on a baking sheet in a single layer.

Roast in the oven for 15-20 minutes, or until slightly browned.

Serve and enjoy.

Nutritional Information:

Calories: 126

Fat: 5g

Carbohydrates: 10g

Protein: 11g

Greek Yogurt and Berry Parfait:

Ingredients:

1 cup of Greek yoghurt

1 cup of mixed berries (e.g. blueberries, strawberries, raspberries)

1/4 cup of granola

Instructions:

Layer the Greek yoghurt, mixed berries, and granola in a glass.

Repeat the layers until all ingredients are used up.

Serve and enjoy.

Nutritional Information:

Calories: 267

Fat: 6g

Carbohydrates: 36g

Protein: 19g

Baked Zucchini Chips:

Ingredients:

2 medium-sized zucchinis, thinly sliced

1 egg

1/2 cup of breadcrumbs

1 tsp garlic powder

Salt and pepper to taste

Instructions:

Preheat oven to 425°F (218°C).

Beat the egg in a small bowl.

In a separate bowl, mix the breadcrumbs, garlic powder, salt, and pepper.

Dip the zucchini slices into the egg mixture, then into the breadcrumb mixture.

Place the coated zucchini slices on a baking sheet in a single layer.

Bake in the oven for 20-25 minutes, or until crispy.

Serve and enjoy.

Nutritional Information:

Calories: 133

Fat: 3g

Carbohydrates: 20g

Protein: 7g

Apple Slices with Almond Butter:

Ingredients:

1 medium-sized apple, sliced

2 tbsp almond butter

Instructions:

Spread almond butter on each apple slice.

Serve and enjoy.

Nutritional Information:

Calories: 188

Fat: 10g

Carbohydrates: 24g

Protein: 4g

Carrots and Hummus:

Ingredients:

1 cup of baby carrots

2 tbsp of hummus

Instructions:

Dip the baby carrots into the hummus.

Serve and enjoy.

Nutritional Information:

Calories: 85

Fat: 4g

Carbohydrates: 11g

Protein: 3g

Cottage Cheese and Berries

Ingredients:

1/2 cup of low-fat cottage cheese

1/2 cup of mixed berries (e.g., blueberries, raspberries, strawberries)

1 tablespoon of honey (optional)

Instructions:

In a small bowl, mix the cottage cheese and berries.

Drizzle with honey (if using) and serve immediately.

Nutritional information per serving:

Calories: 107 kcal

Fat: 1 g

Carbohydrates: 16 g

Fibre: 3 g

Protein: 11 g

Baked Apple Chips

Ingredients:

2 medium apples, cored and thinly sliced

1 tablespoon of cinnamon

Instructions:

Preheat the oven to 200°F (95°C).

Line a baking sheet with parchment paper and arrange the apple slices on it.

Sprinkle the cinnamon evenly over the apple slices.

Bake for 1 1/2 to 2 hours, or until the apple slices are crisp and dry.

Let cool completely before serving.

Nutritional information per serving (1/2 cup):

Calories: 49 kcal

Fat: 0 g

Carbohydrates: 13 g

Fibre: 3 g

Protein: 0 g

Greek Yogurt and Granola

Ingredients:

1/2 cup of plain Greek yoghurt

1/4 cup of granola

1/4 cup of mixed berries (e.g., blueberries, raspberries, strawberries)

Instructions:

In a bowl, layer the yoghurt, granola, and mixed berries.

Serve immediately.

Nutritional information per serving:

Calories: 195 kcal

Fat: 6 g

Carbohydrates:

Apple Cinnamon Yogurt Parfait

Ingredients:

1 medium apple, chopped

1/2 cup non-fat Greek yoghurt

1/4 cup rolled oats

1 tablespoon honey

1/2 teaspoon cinnamon

Instructions:

In a small bowl, mix the Greek yoghurt, honey, and cinnamon.

In a separate bowl, combine the chopped apple and rolled oats.

Layer the apple and oat mixture with the yoghurt mixture in a glass or bowl.

Serve immediately.

Nutritional Information:

Calories: 224

Protein: 15g

Carbohydrates: 43g

Fat: 1g

Fibre: 6g

Sugar: 25g

Roasted Chickpeas

Ingredients:

1 can chickpeas, drained and rinsed

1 tablespoon olive oil

1 teaspoon garlic powder

1 teaspoon paprika

1/2 teaspoon salt

Instructions:

Preheat oven to 400°F.

Rinse and drain the chickpeas, and pat dry with a paper towel.

In a bowl, mix the chickpeas, olive oil, garlic powder, paprika, and salt.

Spread the chickpeas out on a baking sheet in a single layer.

Roast in the oven for 20-30 minutes, or until crispy.

Allow cooling before serving.

Nutritional Information:

Calories: 151

Protein: 6g

Carbohydrates: 22g

Fat: 5g

Fibre: 6g

Sugar: 0g

Dessert Recipes

Here are some healthy Noom diet dessert recipes for seniors:

Banana Oatmeal Cookies

Ingredients:

2 ripe bananas, mashed

1 1/2 cups rolled oats

1/4 cup almond butter

1/4 cup honey

1 tsp vanilla extract

1/2 tsp ground cinnamon

1/4 tsp salt

Instructions:

Preheat the oven to 350°F and line a baking sheet with parchment paper.

In a large mixing bowl, combine all the ingredients and mix well.

Using a cookie scoop, drop the dough onto the prepared baking sheet, spacing them apart.

Bake for 15-20 minutes or until golden brown.

Let the cookies cool completely on the baking sheet before serving.

Nutritional information per serving (1 cookie):

Calories: 96

Fat: 3.5g

Carbohydrates: 15g

Fibre: 2g

Protein: 2g

Berry and Yogurt Parfait

Ingredients:

1 cup plain Greek yoghurt

1/2 cup mixed berries (such as strawberries, blueberries, and raspberries)

1/4 cup granola

1 tsp honey

Instructions:

In a small mixing bowl, mix the yoghurt and honey.

In a separate serving dish, layer the mixed berries, followed by the yoghurt mixture, and then the granola.

Repeat the layers until all ingredients are used up.

Serve immediately or chill in the refrigerator until ready to serve.

Nutritional information per serving:

Calories: 210

Fat: 6g

Carbohydrates: 28g

Fibre: 3g

Protein: 14g

Baked Apples with Cinnamon and Almonds

Ingredients:

2 medium apples, cored and sliced

2 tbsp chopped almonds

1 tbsp honey

1 tsp ground cinnamon

Instructions:

Preheat the oven to 375°F.

In a small mixing bowl, mix the chopped almonds, honey, and cinnamon.

Stuff each apple slice with the almond mixture and place it on a baking dish.

Bake for 20-25 minutes or until the apples are tender.

Let the baked apples cool for a few minutes before serving.

Nutritional information per serving:

Calories: 136

Fat: 3g

Carbohydrates: 28g

Fibre: 5g

Protein: 2g

Berry and Yogurt Parfait

Ingredients:

1 cup mixed berries (strawberries, blueberries, raspberries)

1 cup low-fat plain Greek yoghurt

1/4 cup granola

1 tablespoon honey

Instructions:

In a small bowl, mix the yogurt and honey.

In a glass or bowl, layer the berries, yoghurt mixture, and granola.

Repeat until all ingredients are used.

Serve and enjoy!

Nutritional Information (per serving):

Calories: 225

Fat: 4g

Carbohydrates: 35g

Protein: 16g

Fibre: 6g

Baked Apples with Cinnamon and Walnuts

Ingredients:

2 apples, cored

1/4 cup chopped walnuts

1 tablespoon honey

1/2 teaspoon ground cinnamon

Instructions:

Preheat the oven to 375°F (190°C).

Place the cored apples in a baking dish.

In a small bowl, mix the walnuts, honey, and
 cinnamon.

Spoon the walnut mixture into the apples.

Bake for 20-25 minutes, until the apples are tender
 and the topping is golden brown.

Serve warm and enjoy!

Nutritional Information (per serving):

Calories: 200

Fat: 9g

Carbohydrates: 30g

Protein: 3g

Fibre: 6g

Chocolate Banana Smoothie

Ingredients:

1 banana, peeled

1 cup unsweetened almond milk

2 tablespoons unsweetened cocoa powder

1 tablespoon honey

Instructions:

In a blender, combine the banana, almond milk, cocoa powder, and honey.

Blend until smooth and creamy.

Pour into a glass and enjoy!

Nutritional Information (per serving):

Calories: 160

Fat: 4g

Carbohydrates: 31g

Protein: 4g

Fibre: 7g

Vanilla Chia Pudding

Ingredients:

1 cup unsweetened almond milk

1/4 cup chia seeds

1/2 teaspoon vanilla extract

1 tablespoon honey

Instructions:

In a bowl, whisk together the almond milk, chia seeds, vanilla extract, and honey.

Cover and refrigerate for at least 2 hours or overnight.

Serve and enjoy!

Nutritional Information (per serving):

Calories: 180

Fat: 9g

Carbohydrates: 18g

Protein: 6g / Fibre: 12g

Peanut Butter Banana Bites

Ingredients:

1 banana, sliced

2 tablespoons natural peanut butter

1/4 cup granola

Instructions:

Spread each banana slice with a small amount of peanut butter.

Sprinkle with granola.

Serve and enjoy!

Nutritional Information (per serving):

Calories: 170

Fat: 7

Baked Apple Slices

Ingredients:

2 apples, cored and sliced

1 tbsp honey

1 tsp cinnamon

1/4 tsp nutmeg

Instructions:

Preheat the oven to 375°F.

Arrange the apple slices in a single layer on a baking sheet.

Drizzle honey over the apple slices.

Sprinkle cinnamon and nutmeg over the apple slices.

Bake for 15-20 minutes or until the apples are soft and golden brown.

Nutrition Information (per serving):

Calories: 102

Protein: 0.5g

Fat: 0.3g

Carbohydrates: 27g

Fibre: 4g

Sugar: 21g

Sodium: 0mg

Chocolate Chia Pudding

Ingredients:

1/4 cup chia seeds

1 cup unsweetened almond milk

2 tbsp unsweetened cocoa powder

2 tbsp maple syrup

Instructions:

In a bowl, mix the chia seeds and almond milk. Let it sit for 10 minutes.

Add the cocoa powder and maple syrup to the bowl and mix well.

Cover the bowl with plastic wrap and refrigerate for at least 2 hours or overnight.

Serve the chocolate chia pudding topped with fresh berries or chopped nuts.

Nutrition Information (per serving):

Calories: 173

Protein: 5g

Fat: 10g

Carbohydrates: 22g

Fibre: 12g

Sugar: 7g / Sodium: 79mg

CHAPTER FOUR

MEAL PLANNING FOR THE NOOM DIET

How to Plan Your Weekly Meals

Meal planning for the week can help you keep on track with the Noom diet and ensure you are reaching your nutritional needs. Here are some meal-planning strategies to get you started:

1. **Take stock of your Pantry and Refrigerator:** Before you begin preparing your meals, check to see what items you currently have on hand. This will assist you in avoiding needless purchases and reducing food waste.

2. **Plan your Meals for the Week:** Depending on your nutritional needs and preferences, plan your meals for the week. Including a variety of proteins, complete grains, fruits, and vegetables in your meals might be beneficial.

3. **Create a Grocery List:** Once you've settled on your meals, make a list of all the ingredients you'll need.

4. **Shop for Groceries:** Go to the grocery shop or get your food online. Strive to stick to your shopping list and prevent impulse purchases.

5. **Prepare your Ingredients:** Once you've gathered all of your ingredients, prepare any that can be made ahead of time. This includes washing and slicing veggies as well as preparing grains.

Prepare your meals and keep them in the refrigerator or freezer for convenient access throughout the week. Preparing snacks ahead of time, such as chopping up fruit or preparing energy balls, is also an option.

You may save time and minimize stress during the week by preparing your meals ahead of time while remaining on track with your Noom diet objectives.

Sample meal plans for seniors on the Noom Diet

Week 1:

Monday

Breakfast: Greek yoghurt with mixed berries and chopped almonds

Lunch: Lentil soup with a mixed green salad and whole wheat pita bread

Dinner: Baked salmon with roasted Brussels sprouts and sweet potato wedges

Tuesday

Breakfast: Avocado toast on whole grain bread with a side of fresh fruit

Lunch: Grilled chicken salad with mixed greens, cherry tomatoes, and cucumber

Dinner: Quinoa and vegetable stir-fry

Wednesday

Breakfast: Oatmeal with sliced banana and chopped walnuts

Lunch: Whole grain wrap with turkey, avocado, tomato, and lettuce

Dinner: Vegetable lasagna with a side of garlic bread

Thursday

Breakfast: Scrambled eggs with spinach and tomatoes on whole wheat toast

Lunch: Roasted vegetable and chickpea bowl

Dinner: Grilled shrimp skewers with a side of grilled zucchini and brown rice

Friday

Breakfast: Protein smoothie with banana, almond milk, and spinach

Lunch: Whole grain pasta salad with mixed vegetables and a side of fruit

Dinner: Beef and broccoli stir-fried with brown rice

Saturday

Breakfast: Whole grain waffles with fresh fruit and a dollop of Greek yoghurt

Lunch: Grilled portobello mushroom burger on a whole grain bun with a side of sweet potato fries

Dinner: Roasted chicken with mixed vegetables and quinoa

Sunday

Breakfast: Veggie omelette with a side of whole-grain toast

Lunch: Chicken and vegetable kebabs with a side of tabbouleh

Dinner: Grilled flank steak with a side of roasted root vegetables

Week 2:

Monday

Breakfast: Greek yoghurt with sliced strawberries and honey

Snack: Apple slices with almond butter

Lunch: Tomato and mozzarella salad with basil and balsamic glaze

Snack: Roasted chickpeas

Dinner: Grilled salmon with asparagus and quinoa

Tuesday

Breakfast: Egg white omelette with spinach, mushrooms, and feta cheese

Snack: Carrot sticks with hummus

Lunch: Turkey and avocado wrap with mixed greens

Snack: Cottage cheese with pineapple chunks

Dinner: Turkey chilli with mixed vegetables and brown rice

Wednesday

Breakfast: Banana and peanut butter smoothie

Snack: Trail mix with nuts and dried fruit

Lunch: Lentil soup with whole-grain bread

Snack: Baby carrots with ranch dressing

Dinner: Spaghetti squash with turkey meatballs and marinara sauce

Thursday

Breakfast: Overnight oats with almond milk, berries, and chia seeds

Snack: Roasted edamame

Lunch: Grilled chicken salad with mixed greens and honey mustard dressing

Snack: Hard-boiled egg

Dinner: Grilled sirloin steak with roasted Brussels sprouts and sweet potato

Friday

Breakfast: Veggie omelette with spinach, tomatoes, and onions

Snack: Fresh berries with whipped cream

Lunch: Tuna salad with mixed greens and whole-grain crackers

Snack: Air-popped popcorn

Dinner: Grilled shrimp with zucchini noodles and pesto sauce

Saturday

Breakfast: Whole-grain pancakes with sliced banana and maple syrup

Snack: Greek yoghurt with honey and mixed nuts

Lunch: Grilled chicken wrap with mixed vegetables and hummus

Snack: Cucumber slices with tzatziki sauce

Dinner: Baked salmon with roasted asparagus and quinoa

Sunday

Breakfast: Sweet potato hash with scrambled eggs and turkey sausage

Snack: Sliced pear with almond butter

Lunch: Grilled portobello mushroom burger with avocado and tomato

Snack: Roasted pumpkin seeds

Dinner: Stuffed bell peppers with ground turkey and brown rice

Week 3:

Monday

Breakfast: Greek yoghurt with mixed berries and chopped almonds

Lunch: Lentil soup with a mixed green salad and whole wheat pita bread

Dinner: Baked salmon with roasted asparagus and brown rice

Tuesday

Breakfast: Avocado toast on whole grain bread with a side of fresh fruit

Lunch: Grilled chicken salad with mixed greens, cherry tomatoes, and cucumber

Dinner: Quinoa and black bean bowl

Wednesday

Breakfast: Oatmeal with sliced banana and chopped walnuts

Lunch: Whole grain wrap with turkey, avocado, tomato, and lettuce

Dinner: Vegetable curry with brown rice

Thursday

Breakfast: Scrambled eggs with spinach and tomatoes on whole wheat toast

Lunch: Roasted vegetable and quinoa bowl

Dinner: Grilled fish tacos with a side of salsa and avocado

Friday

Breakfast: Protein smoothie with banana, almond milk, and spinach

Lunch: Whole grain pasta salad with mixed vegetables and a side of fruit

Dinner: Turkey and vegetable chilli with a side of cornbread

Saturday

Breakfast: Whole grain pancakes with fresh fruit and a dollop of Greek yoghurt

Lunch: Grilled portobello mushroom burger on a whole grain bun with a side of roasted sweet potatoes

Dinner: Grilled chicken with mixed vegetables and sweet potato mash

Sunday

Breakfast: Veggie omelette with a side of whole-grain toast

Lunch: Grilled vegetable and hummus wrap with a side of tabbouleh

Dinner: Beef and vegetable stir-fry with brown rice

Week 4:

Monday

Breakfast: Greek yoghurt with fresh berries and chia seeds

Snack: Sliced cucumbers with hummus

Lunch: Turkey and avocado sandwich on whole wheat bread, side of baby carrots

Snack: Apple slices with almond butter

Dinner: Baked salmon with roasted asparagus and sweet potato

Tuesday

Breakfast: Quinoa breakfast bowl with banana, almond milk, and cinnamon

Snack: Rice cakes with almond butter and sliced banana

Lunch: Tuna salad with mixed greens and cherry tomatoes

Snack: Greek yoghurt with honey and granola

Dinner: Stuffed bell peppers with ground turkey and quinoa

Wednesday

Breakfast: Smoothie with spinach, banana, almond milk, and protein powder

Snack: Sliced cucumbers with tzatziki dip

Lunch: Lentil and vegetable soup

Snack: Trail mix with almonds, cashews, and dried cranberries

Dinner: Grilled chicken with roasted broccoli and cauliflower rice

Thursday

Breakfast: Oatmeal with fresh berries and sliced almonds

Snack: Apple slices with almond butter

Lunch: Grilled shrimp salad with mixed greens, cucumber, and cherry tomatoes

Snack: Greek yoghurt with honey and fresh fruit

Dinner: Baked tofu with stir-fried vegetables and brown rice

Friday

Breakfast: Scrambled eggs with sautéed mushrooms and spinach

Snack: Rice cakes with almond butter and sliced banana

Lunch: Chicken and vegetable stir-fry with brown rice

Snack: Sliced bell peppers with hummus

Dinner: Grilled salmon with roasted Brussels sprouts and sweet potato

Saturday

Breakfast: Smoothie with banana, almond milk, and protein powder

Snack: Sliced cucumbers with tzatziki dip

Lunch: Turkey and vegetable wrap on a whole wheat tortilla

Snack: Trail mix with almonds, cashews, and dried cranberries

Dinner: Baked chicken with roasted asparagus and quinoa

Sunday

Breakfast: Greek yoghurt with fresh berries and chia seeds

Snack: Rice cakes with almond butter and sliced banana

Lunch: Lentil and vegetable soup

Snack: Sliced apples with almond butter

Dinner: Grilled shrimp with roasted broccoli and cauliflower rice

Tips for Grocery Shopping and Meal Prep

Here are some tips for grocery shopping and meal prep on the Noom diet for seniors:

Make a Grocery List: Before heading to the store, create a list of the ingredients you need for your meal plan. This will help you stay on track and avoid impulse purchases.

Shop the Perimeter: Stick to the outer aisles of the grocery store, where you will find fresh produce, lean proteins, and dairy products. Avoid processed and packaged foods in the centre aisles.

Buy in bulk: Purchasing items like whole grains, nuts, and seeds in bulk can save you money in the long run. Just make sure to store them properly to maintain freshness.

Prep in Advance: Spend a few hours on the weekend prepping your meals for the week. Chop vegetables, cook grains, and portion out snacks so you can easily grab them throughout the week.

Use meal Prep Containers: Invest in some meal prep containers to store your meals and snacks in. This will make it easy to grab and go throughout the week.

Don't be afraid to freeze: If you make a large batch of a recipe, freeze the leftovers in individual portions for easy meals later on.

Stay organized: Keep your fridge and pantry organized so you can easily find the ingredients you need. This will also help you avoid food waste by keeping track of what you have on hand.

CHAPTER FIVE

NOOM DIET SUCCESS TIPS FOR SENIORS

Staying motivated on the Noom Diet

Staying motivated on the Noom diet can be challenging, especially for seniors who may have been set in their ways of eating for many years. Here are some tips to help seniors stay motivated on the Noom diet:

Set achievable goals: Start with small goals and gradually increase them over time. Setting unrealistic goals can lead to frustration and can discourage seniors from continuing with the diet.

Find a support system: Having a support system can make a big difference in staying motivated. Encourage seniors to find a friend or family member to join them on the Noom diet, or to join a support group or online community.

Celebrate successes: Celebrate the small successes along the way. Whether it's losing a few pounds or sticking to the diet for a week, acknowledge the achievement and use it as motivation to keep going.

Keep it interesting: Variety is key to staying motivated. Encourage seniors to try new recipes and foods, or to mix up their exercise routine to keep things interesting and prevent boredom.

Track progress: Tracking progress can help seniors see how far they've come and keep them motivated to continue. Whether it's using the Noom app or keeping a journal, tracking progress can be a powerful motivator.

Overcoming common challenges and obstacles
Starting a new diet or lifestyle can be challenging, and the Noom diet is no exception. Here are some tips for overcoming common challenges and obstacles while following the Noom diet:

1. **Lack of motivation:** It's normal to experience dips in motivation when starting a new diet. To stay motivated, remind yourself of your reasons for starting the Noom diet, and set achievable goals for yourself. Celebrate your successes, no matter how small they may seem.

2. **Cravings:** It's common to experience cravings for unhealthy foods, especially in the early stages of the diet. To combat this, try keeping healthy snacks on hand, such as fruit or veggies, and allow yourself the occasional indulgence in moderation.

3. **Eating out:** Eating out can be a challenge when following a specific diet. To make healthier choices when eating out, do some research on restaurant menus ahead of time, and opt for grilled or roasted options rather than fried or breaded dishes.

4. **Social pressure:** Social pressure to indulge in unhealthy foods can be a challenge. To overcome this, be honest with your friends and family about your dietary goals, and suggest healthier options for group meals or events.

5. **Plateaus:** It's common to experience weight loss plateaus when following a diet. To overcome this, mix up your exercise routine, try new healthy recipes, and focus on non-scale victories, such as increased energy levels or improved sleep quality.

Remember, the Noom diet is about making sustainable, long-term lifestyle changes. Be patient with yourself, and celebrate your progress along the way.

Lifestyle changes to support your weight loss goals
Making lifestyle changes is an important part of the Noom diet plan for seniors. While the diet focuses on making healthier food choices and portion control, it

also emphasizes the importance of making lasting changes to support weight loss goals.

Here are some lifestyle changes that can support your weight loss efforts:

Regular Exercise: Physical activity is an essential part of any weight loss plan. It not only helps to burn calories but also strengthens muscles, improves flexibility, and reduces the risk of chronic diseases. Aim for at least 30 minutes of moderate-intensity exercise, such as brisk walking or cycling, five days a week.

Adequate sleep: Getting enough sleep is crucial for weight loss success. Sleep deprivation can disrupt hormones that regulate hunger and metabolism, leading to increased appetite and weight gain. Aim for seven to eight hours of sleep per night.

Stress management: Chronic stress can trigger overeating and lead to weight gain. Finding healthy ways to manage stress, such as meditation, deep breathing, or yoga, can help prevent emotional eating.

Mindful eating: Mindful eating involves paying attention to your food and eating slowly, without distractions. This can help you tune into your body's hunger and fullness signals, and make better food choices.

Hydration: Drinking enough water is essential for weight loss success. Aim for at least eight glasses of water per day, and limit sugary drinks.

By making these lifestyle changes and incorporating the Noom diet plan, seniors can not only lose weight but also improve their overall health and well-being. It's important to remember that making lasting changes takes time and effort, but the benefits are worth it.

Conclusion

In conclusion, the Noom diet is a lifestyle change that can help seniors achieve their weight loss goals. By focusing on nutrient-dense, low-calorie foods and creating healthy habits, seniors can improve their overall health and well-being. With colour-coded food categories, meal planning, and smart grocery shopping, seniors can enjoy a variety of delicious and satisfying meals on the Noom diet. While there may be some challenges and obstacles along the way, staying motivated and committed to the program can lead to long-term success. Remember, small changes can make a big difference, and by making healthy choices every day, seniors can achieve their weight loss and wellness goals.

Appendix: Noom Diet Food List

Here is an appendix of the Noom diet food list:

Green Foods:

Non-starchy vegetables (broccoli, cauliflower, spinach, kale, etc.)

Whole grains (brown rice, quinoa, barley, etc.)

Low-fat dairy (milk, cheese, yoghurt)

Fresh fruit (berries, apples, oranges, etc.)

Lean proteins (chicken breast, turkey, fish, tofu, legumes, etc.)

Healthy fats (avocado, nuts, seeds, olive oil)

Yellow Foods:

Starchy vegetables (potatoes, corn, peas, etc.)

Whole grain bread and pasta

Higher-fat dairy (butter, full-fat cheese)

Tropical fruits (banana, mango, pineapple)

Lean red meats (beef, pork)

Processed meats (bacon, sausage, deli meat)

Red Foods:

Processed snacks (chips, crackers, cookies, etc.)

Fried foods (fast food, fried chicken, etc.)

Sugary drinks (soda, sports drinks, energy drinks, etc.)

High-fat dairy (ice cream, cream cheese, whipped cream)

Red meats (beef, pork)

Sweets and candy (chocolate, candy bars, etc.)

It is important to note that Noom does not completely restrict any food groups, but rather emphasizes portion control and balance. The program encourages users to consume mostly green foods, limit yellow foods, and only consume red foods in moderation. By following these guidelines, seniors can enjoy a well-rounded and nutritious diet while still achieving their weight loss goals.

Glossary

Here are some common terms related to the Noom diet:

Noom Coach: An app-based weight loss program that helps users achieve their weight loss goals through personalized coaching, meal tracking, and exercise logging.

Calorie Density: The number of calories per gram of food. Foods with high-calorie density have more calories per gram than foods with low-calorie density.

Green Foods: These are low-calorie-density foods, which means they have fewer calories per gram than yellow or red foods. Examples include fruits, vegetables, whole grains, and lean proteins.

Yellow Foods: These are moderate-calorie-density foods that should be eaten in moderation. Examples include whole wheat bread, eggs, and low-fat dairy products.

Red Foods: These are high-calorie-density foods that should be limited. Examples include processed foods, fried foods, and sugary drinks.

Portion Control: The practice of eating a specific amount of food at each meal, often measured in serving sizes.

Mindful Eating: The practice of paying attention to your body's hunger cues and eating slowly and without distractions, such as TV or phone.

Meal Planning: The practice of prepping and planning your meals ahead of time to ensure you have healthy options on hand.

Meal Prep: The act of preparing meals in advance, such as cooking food in batches and storing it for later use.

Plate Method: A method of portion control where half of your plate is filled with non-starchy vegetables, one-quarter with lean protein, and one-quarter with whole grains or starchy vegetables.

Made in United States
North Haven, CT
17 April 2023

35538192R00063